The Hidden Dangers of Leaky Gut Syndrome:

What Your Doctor Won't Tell You

I0423277

Teresa Banks

Disclaimer

This book is intended for informational and educational purposes only. Nothing in this book should be taken as medical advice. Before you embark on any new health program, consult your personal physician or natural health care practitioner.

Table of Contents

Introduction

Wouldn't it be great if you could experience health, vitality, and energy again? What someone tells you that your autoimmune disease can be cured? Imagine yourself pain-free and to free yourself from a chronic disorder irritable bowel syndrome, or even alleviate the symptoms of your rheumatoid arthritis.

What I tell you that I have the "cure" easing these symptoms? Would you be willing to find out more about it? You're probably nodding your hear as you read this. Many other people who are suffering will also agree with you.

But you think to yourself, "if there were such a solution, what would it be and why haven't I heard about it before? Why hasn't my doctor told me about it?"

Those are very legitimate questions.

It is possible that your doctor may never have heard of this syndrome. Most allopathic doctors don't know about it. And those who have don't give too much attention in the syndrome. They might not believe that it's a real health concern.

You must find a doctor or a specialist who are knowledgeable in this condition. But this is not easy and most conventional doctors won't even suspect this disorder.

For this reason alone, it's nearly impossible to estimate with any accuracy how many people are affected with this problem. Some alternate health professionals have theorized the number affected could even be in the millions worldwide.

Even many professionals who do recognize and diagnose this syndrome usually would suspect a wide-ranging and varied assortment of unrelated symptoms to it. The symptoms can range from gluten intolerance, food allergies and sensitivities, muscle cramps, fibromyalgia, and even acne.

Doctors failing to recognize this disorder doesn't make it any less real. The truth is that you've been suffering for too long . . . visiting far too many specialists . . . and enduring far too many different proposed remedies that don't work.

Relief . . .

I don't have to tell you what the consequences of all this misinformation and ignorance are; you already know it, because you're the one living with it. You've found no relief and you still have the same pain you did when you first started. Only perhaps now you've been the recipient of untold numbers of prescription medications that don't work.

Not to add salt to the wound, but natural health care specialists say that one of the causes of leaky gut syndrome is . . . well, overuse of prescription medications -- specifically antibiotics. Ouch! Isn't it ironic? In your attempt to discover relief, you have been unwittingly making your condition even worse.

So, what to do then?

You might be losing hope and ready to give up feeling like there's no hope of you ever discovering if your problem is -- underneath it all -- due to leaky gut syndrome.

Don't give up, not just yet. That's what this book is all about. It's your personal resource and reference manual to help you understand the complexity of leaky gut syndrome. This book also contains many useful advice (that you can start using nearly immediately) to help you identify and overcome this complex health concern that you've having for much too long.

This book doesn't just detailed what leaky gut is and what causes it, but I've even devoted a chapter to how your personal health care provider goes about making definitive, accurate diagnosis.

Diagnosis: You Can't Heal if You Can't Pin Point It!

Once you are diagnosed correctly, then leaky gut becomes far less mysterious and threatening. An accurate diagnosis also provides you with the beginnings of the possibility of an effective treatment.

All these can provide you with something you haven't felt, I suspect, in a long time: hope.

Once you are correctly diagnosed that you're suffering from leaky gut, you can take the necessary steps to overcome it. I will provide you with a variety of ways that you can start healing your body. From diet to dietary supplements to herbs and beyond, you can choose the solutions that work for your specific, individual health problems.

Before You Begin

Before you get excited and jumping into a program, you need to consult a health care provider. This means finding a reliable naturopathic doctor to guide you, or you may need to visit a good, reputable integrated medical clinic.

But if you've truly been suffering with what turns out to be leaky gut, you need to discover relief -- and quickly. Reading this book will be well worth your time.

Imagine . . . living pain free and symptom free again!

What is leaky gut syndrome?

It won't be a surprise if your first thought is that there couldn't possibly be a health condition named **leaky gut syndrome (LGS)**. But let me assure you, despite the allopathic medical community's refusal to acknowledge leaky gut, many natural health care practitioners are extremely aware of it.

It is also known by a more professional-sounding name: increased intestinal permeability.

Leaky gut syndrome happens when the lining of your intestine becomes inflamed, and then irritation occurs. When this occurs, the permeability of the lining is compromised. This means that the lining, which normally acts like a fortress wall allowing nothing to pass through, fails to do its job properly.

This literally means your gut "leaks"; allowing bacteria and other toxins, as well as proteins and fats that aren't completely digested, to escape into your bloodstream.

As your body detects these toxins, it triggers an autoimmune reaction in which the immune system attacks your own cells. And this can eventually cause a couple gastrointestinal problems. This can come in a form of abdominal bloating, excess gas, and cramps.

But there are other ways this situation can affect your body as well:

- Fatigue
- Food sensitivities
- Joint pain

Many of the symptoms show up in a variety of forms and conditions. They are also considered disorders and diseases in and of themselves. Doctors and we don't usually link them to leaky gut syndrome. Listed below are just a handful of these symptoms:

- Alcohol use
- Autoimmune diseases
- Candida
- Certain medications
- Chronic constipation
- Chronic stress
- Environmental toxins
- Excessive consumption of processed foods
- Food sensitivities
- Low- fiber diet

- Low-stomach acid
- Nutritional deficiencies
- Severe burns

Most of the time we consider these symptoms as disorders. We treat them, but don't realize why they exist to begin with. The truth of the matter is that as the toxins get into your blood, they eventually affect other parts of your body. Many of which are still banding together trying hard to keep you healthy.

Leaky gut syndrome and your liver

Your **liver** is among the first organs to be affected. The more toxins that enter your system, the more your liver works at excreting them. This keeps your organ very active – too active. If left untreated, the liver gets overloaded and can no longer detoxify these materials. As a result, the minerals and toxins returned to the blood to circulate.

Maintenance of chemical homeostasis is one of the tasks our blood performs. Through this mechanism, your body attempts to maintain an internal stability. It skillfully coordinates the responses of various actions of different organs throughout your system. If for any reason the balance is disturbed, the poisonous chemicals and some physical debris get delivered to into what's called the tissue matrix.

Lymph system

Once this imbalance occurs, that's when another organ jumps into action: your **lymph system**. It will try to maintain a healthy balance. It's a vital part of your immune system.

Your lymphatic system will try to collect and then neutralize these toxins, but it's not always successful. When this happens, it then puts the burden on liver and the tissue matrix, which have the potential to turn toxic.

It will take some time, but what was initially just a "gut-barrier" issue has escalated into tissue toxicity. And this in turn can trigger a domino effect of chain reaction of other problems. If your tissue environment is compromised, bacteria grow.

Adding to those problems, the lymph fluids in your body accumulate causing lymphatic swelling. You'll soon realize the presence of inflammation in your body. This swelling is what causes the multitude of possible symptoms, some of which go unexplained.

The consequences of toxin build up

If too many toxins accumulate in your body, the immune system exhausts itself working against them. This process also depletes your immune system.

Why does it affect the immune system? You wonder. It has been a fact not known to many that 70% of your immune system is actually located in and around your digestive system.

This portion of the system is called gut-associated lymphatic tissues, or GALT. These tissues are located in the lining of the digestive tract and in the intestinal mucus.

What happens when the liver is overworked?

Toxin buildup will literally overwhelm your liver, leaving it unable to process everything efficiently. When this happens, the liver then turns to your immune system for help. Unfortunately, in turn your immune response is stressed, unable to act properly like it should.

Bacteria will then accumulate to unhealthy levels, and this opens the door for opportunistic infections to appear. These infections will be infections you normally wouldn't develop. They are able to sneak in because of the severely weakened state of your immune system.

Your **adrenal glands** will be the next organ that will be affected by this unwanted bacteria. They are two small glands sitting atop each of your kidneys. Your adrenal glands are vital in resisting infections. Prolonged presence of leaky gut syndrome will eventually reduce the healthy function of these glands as well.

As the syndrome continues undetected, cortisol levels drop. When this happens, another condition called adrenal exhaustion occurs. Your adrenal glands are "tired" or "over-worked". This can be easily tested by measuring your cortisol output, the hormone the adrenal glands produce.

A few of the symptoms indicating you may be experiencing adrenal fatigue include:

- Exhaustion
- Sleep that doesn't refresh you
- Inability to cope with stress
- Difficulty concentrating
- Poor digestion

How to spot leaky gut syndrome

Now that, at least in general terms, you have understood how the syndrome develops, hopefully you have a greater appreciation for how all the parts of your body work together to help fight off disease and keeping you healthy.

It's not a surprise if you discover that leaky gut syndrome can manifest itself in any number of ways in your system. While you can't call these "symptoms," they are indeed real health conditions. But the underlying cause of these conditions may very well be the presence of leaky gut syndrome.

I will discuss some of the factors that can cause leaky gut syndrome in the next chapter. Knowing what cause and trigger this syndrome will help you take action to remedy it.

The Causes of Leaky Gut Syndrome that No One Talks About

What causes it?

I wish there is an answer to that question, but there isn't. In fact, there are a huge number of possible causes of this syndrome. And there are "hidden" causes that no one talks about.

So, if you're hoping and waiting for your health care provider to hand over one cause on a silver platter -- well, forget about it. More often than not discovering the cause is sometimes the most difficult part of treating the syndrome.

No one knows your body better than you. You know your health habits. And armed with this intimate information, when you're presented with a list of possible hidden causes

---

you may be able to separate the most probable causes first and check them out.

Below are just a few of the more common causes of this syndrome:

- Chronic use of NSAIDs
- Dysbiosis
- Candida
- Cancer therapy
- Chronic stress
- Environmental toxins
- Diet
- Aging
- Endotoxins
- AIDS
- Gastrointestinal disease
- Immune system overload
- Lack of Secretory IgA
- Abuse of alcohol
- Trauma
- Chronic infections

NSAIDs as a cause

We live in a time and age that practically demands instant gratification. To some people, that means piling huge amounts of pleasure on themselves.

This also means that when they feel pain, they want it gone as soon as possible. This is the reason why many people immediately opt for a class of pain medications commonly known by its initials, **NSAID** (non-steroidal anti-inflammatory drugs). They include aspirin, naproxen, and ibuprofen.

These medications are different than steroids, which have similar anti-inflammatory effects on the body. All of the NSAIDs are over-the-counter medication, and can be bought without a doctor's prescription.

Most people depend on these types of drugs in order to relieve all types of pain, from a headache to chronic arthritis. Few of us, though, give any real thought to their possible side effects. The development of leaky gut syndrome is one of them.

NSAIDs and prostaglandins

NSAIDs are known for their ability to block tiny messengers known as **prostaglandins**. As you take NSAIDs, they circulate throughout your body and block pain and inflammation. But that's all they do.

There is another job that they do: they're charged with healing and repairing your body! When you take an NSAID, it blocks the pain and giving yourself much-needed relief you are craving. But you are also effectively blocking any healing or repair process that needs to be performed.

That's right...even though they do a great job in what they're supposed to do, over-the-counter medication indiscriminately blocks all of the transmitters.

How the digestive tract repairs itself

The digestive tract repairs and replaces itself every 3-5 days. So you can see how the extended use of NSAIDs blocks the process of reparation. When this process is blocked for an extended period of time, the lining of the tract eventually weakens, becomes inflamed, and then leaks. And the result is...yes, you have a leaky gut syndrome!

In addition, prolonged use of NSAIDs raises your risk of developing ulcers of the stomach and the duodenum.

There are other significantly good reasons why you would like to reduce your dependency on them. This type of medication causes bleeding, damage to the mucus membranes of your intestines, and gastrointestinal inflammation.

In addition to what already mentioned, NSAID use can lead to colitis and relapses of ulcerative colitis. Who knew that the easily accessible, almost ubiquitous pills everyone takes with barely a second thought could be so potentially troublesome?

Dysbiosis

Most likely, you've probably never heard of dysbiosis. The word was created by Dr. Eli Metchnikoff, a 1908 Nobel Prize winner for his work on friendly bacterial flora.

It's important to keep a good balance between the harmful (pathogenic bacteria) and the helpful bacteria, often called flora.

When your body contains more of the harmful than friendly bacteria, an imbalance occurs. This state is called dysbiosis. It's derived from the word symbiosis, which means "living in harmony" and the prefix dys which means "not."

It has been discovered by Dr. Metchnikoff that the natural bacteria of yogurt can prevent and actually reverse bacterial infections. He also revealed that the bacteria in yogurt has the ability to remove quite a few organisms that cause diseases. In addition, the yogurt bacteria content could also reduce the amount of accompanying toxins.

With the widely used of antibiotics and immunizations, this research seemed far less important and outdated. Given the state of modern medicine at the turn of the 20th century, this represented an amazing advance in the treatment of bacterial infections.

There are many new laboratory testing and corresponding research being done, and this has created a revival in the interest of the topic.

Microbes and your health

There are microbes being discovered that don't belong in the digestive tract. Why is this important to know? The microbes very often form chemicals toxic to the cells which are located around them. But that's only part of the increase in interest. These microbes can also be a source of poison to you.

Having a lot of these microbes puts the lining of your intestines at risk. The likelihood consequence of this is can lead to creations of potentially dangerous substances, including secondary bile acids, amines, phenols ammonia, indoles, and hydrogen sulfide.

Having these substances in your body can injure the brush borders and may damage your intestine lining. The brush borders are the largest manufacturer of digestive enzymes in your small intestine. Eventually the damaged brush borders enzymes (unhealthy) may be absorbed into your bloodstream.

What is frightening is that the damages they're making to your body isn't recognized immediately. After a while they can cause chronic conditions, many of which never get diagnosed.

What exactly causes dysbiosis? As we discussed earlier, it is the overuse of NSAIDs. But the extended use of NSAIDs is only one trigger to the development of the buildup of bad bacteria. We'll discuss the other class of drugs which can trigger this state next.

Antibiotics

Most of us see Antibiotics as the cure for many things. They cure my infections -- all sorts of infections. I get them when I have swollen glands. Well, you get the idea. They're a modern day marvel!

Yes, they do all the beneficial things mentioned above, but that's where the problem comes in. The medical community and most of us have been dependent on this amazing type of medication for just about any ailment. Most patients practically demand some sort of antibiotics when they walk into a doctor's office complaining of an ailment, even if they don't suffer from a bacterial infection. Unfortunately, most doctors will gladly oblige.

When good antibiotics go bad

Try to imagine this: when you put antibiotics in your body, you're potentially disturbing the balance of intestinal microbes. Antibiotics, just like the NSAIDs, really don't discriminate in their attack of bacteria. They kill all kinds of bacteria. The bad and the good!

When this happens, your system may be exposed to resistant bacteria (those that antibiotics can't seem to kill effectively), fungi, parasites, and viruses. A healthy balanced gut usually can keep this array of intruders at bay, thanks to the presence of friendly flora.

When an imbalance occurs and there are more harmful bacteria, the results can be irritation, inflammation and, given enough time, the presence of disease.

The most common microbe to appear because of this imbalance is the yeast infection Candida (a fungus).

Candida and leaky gut syndrome

If you've suffered a Candida infection, then you know how it feels like to have dysbiosis. At least one type of imbalance.

Candida is a fungus that is present in all of us, but usually in small amounts. It can lead to infection when there is an unhealthy amount.

Your strong immune system, a balanced intestinal pH and your friendly flora can easily keep them under control when there are in small amounts.

The Invasion of Candida

If the balance is tilted, the Candida takes advantage by growing and overrunning certain areas of your digestive tract. These fungi create a chemical called acid protease, which "steals" the secretory IgA from the mucus membranes.

And when this happens, the Candida will anchor itself and eventually continue to accumulate on your mucus membrane. This is when infection will occur.

Once anchored and firmly in place, the Candida leaks toxins that leak into the bloodstream. Once they're circulating throughout your body, the toxins destroys your immune system. To make matters worse, they also play havoc with the hormonal balance of your system and even disturb the healthy functioning of your brain!

How about increased food sensitivity?

Antibiotics naturally respond by alerting your immune system to the presence of certain foods which in turn increases your sensitivity to them. Later in this chapter I'll discuss the difference between food sensitivity and a true food allergy. Yes, there is a difference.

This infection can be caused by prolonged use of antibiotics and steroid medications. Many females develop it through the continued use of birth control pills. And still others find that the consumption of alcohol can trigger this condition.

How to tell if you have a Candida infection

So, how can you tell if you have a Candida infection? Is it possible that you are sitting with it right now as you reading this? It's possible. Some of the more obvious symptoms include:

- Abdominal bloating
- Anxiety
- Constipation or Diarrhea (or both!)
- Depression
- Sensitivities to the environment
- Fatigue
- Food sensitivities

- Foggy thought processes

- Insomnia

- Low blood sugar

- Mood swings

- Premenstrual syndrome

- Chronic vaginal infections

- Recurrent bladder infections

- Tinnitus

All those mentioned can indicate other underlying health problems as well as the presence of a yeast infection. And that's exactly why Candida can be difficult to diagnose and goes unnoticed for so long.

Steroid drugs and leaky gut syndrome

Most people, one time or another, have used Steroid drugs. They're used to treat many stubborn lingering health conditions and chronic health problems. They're most effective on allergies, inflammation, and autoimmune diseases. However, prolonged use of steroids eventually weakens your immune system. And yes, you already know this can cause trouble.

A weakened immune system will give way for the development of a fungal infection to take place, not only in your gastrointestinal tract, but in just about every other part of your body.

The Side effects

You might be already dealing with medications to treat some serious disease such as cancer. You're undergoing chemotherapy or radiation treatment. Or maybe both. You don't need any more problems added into your already though life.

The last thing you would like to hear is being told that these same drugs may be triggering the development of leaky gut syndrome. Unfortunately, it's true. Both treatments can possibly disturb the balance of your gastrointestinal tract. That means you may eventually acquire a problem with absorbing foods.

Stress and leaky gut syndrome

Do you know that chronic stress affects your immune system? It does. Stress weakens your ability to fight off infections as well as slows down the healing process of wounds and injuries. When under stress, your body reduces its production of secretory IgA and DHEA, an adrenal hormone that delays the aging process and helps you handle stress.

High stress can also:

- Slows the digestive process,

- Reduces blood flow to your digestive

- Contributes to the manufacturing of toxic metabolites (Metabolites, by the way, are substances crucial to your metabolism.)

It is impossible to avoid stress and it is so much a part of our lives, I've dedicated an entire chapter to various methods that can help you manage the stress in your life. Managing stress may be invaluable to helping you improve your leaky gut syndrome.

How the Environment Affects You

All of us are affected by the environment on a daily basis. Oh, I'm not talking about soaking up the warming rays of the sun, pollens that make you itch or feeling cold from the rain. I'm talking about some serious adverse effects that could be harming your body even as you read this.

All of us are exposed to hundreds of household irritants, environmental chemicals, dangerous chemicals and toxic metals every day. And this constant barrage of exposure is overloading your immune system. It also prevents your system from repairing itself.

One of the things that suffer first is the breaking down of your connective tissue. Soon after that, your body begins lacking in various trace minerals like calcium, potassium, and magnesium.

All these will cause acidosis within your cells and the swelling of tissues and cells.

Your diet as a source of leaky gut syndrome

Hey look, it's a cause of leaky gut syndrome that you can actually control! Your diet. I will not go too deeply into this topic here, because I've devoted an entire chapter to rebalancing your system through changes in your eating habits.

A lack of fiber in your diet can lead to constipation. When you eat a diet that is deficient in fiber, you are effectively promoting a prolonged transit time -- a situation that's not conducive to proper digestion.

The slowing of delivery will hinder your bowel movements and it will also invite toxic byproducts to accumulate and irritate your gut.

Processed foods are one of the worst culprits in causing this disorder. These foods are usually filled with artificial additives, many of which are toxic.

The difference between food sensitivity and allergy

There is a thin line linking food sensitivities and leaky gut syndrome. It's difficult even for the best nutritionists to decide which health problem cropped up first.

Which one came first and caused the other? It's hard to tell, but one thing is fairly certain: the two seem to interlink.

Many individuals confuse food sensitivity with a true food allergy. They are not the same. Surprised? There is no better time to explain the differences than now!

Food allergies: A food allergy is when the body's immune system reacts unusually to specific foods. Allergic reactions are often mild, but they can sometimes be very serious.

The first difference between the two is the reaction time. Food allergies (type 1 or immediate hypersensitivity reaction), trigger the response of certain a specific type of antibody. This antibody bonds to the food antigens and releases substances called cytokines. This will result in a number of allergic symptoms:

- Hives
- Itching
- Runny nose
- Skin rash

Some people may react more seriously such as respiratory distress, the closing your throat, asthma, and even anaphylactic shock.

A life-threatening condition, anaphylactic shock -- or anaphylaxis -- is an extremely serious reaction that affects your entire body. After being exposed to what they are allergic to, let's say, your immune system becomes sensitized to it. Another exposure to it may illicit this allergic reaction.

What's very dangerous about food allergies is the extremely fast response your body has to it. Very often it happens within minutes, which means you must not only be aware of the contact with the allergen immediately, but be ready to act quickly.

Your physician can diagnose food allergies through specific blood testing and patch skin tests.

So do I have a food sensitivity?

It's a possibility. The easiest to differentiate between food sensitivity and food allergy is the reaction time. The first symptom of a food sensitivity is that very often the effects of it are not immediately apparent. This shows up in its medical name delayed hypersensitivity reaction.

It may take hours or even days from the moment you eat the food to the time your reactions surface. But as you can see, it is difficult to pin point what you ate days before that caused your reaction.

Different people react differently to different things – which makes the sensitivity hard to recognize.

Food sensitivity occurs when the food particles escape through the damaged mucosal membranes, and then enters your blood stream.

These food particles are viewed as foreign substances by your body, it then signals your immune system to spring into action. In turn, your liver reacts because it too believes these are toxic. The liver starts the process of breaking them down.

If you don't stop eating these foods, you are increasing the permeability of your intestines. This will continue as a vicious because you'll surely acquire even more food sensitivities over time.

Different people are sensitive to different types of foods, but the following sources account for nearly 80 percent of the adverse reactions: beef, citrus fruits, dairy products, eggs, pork, and wheat.

Perhaps you suspect your health condition -- or multiple conditions -- is caused ultimately by your leaky intestinal lining. Your next move is to visit a physician who believes that this syndrome actually exists. He or she can run you through a battery of diagnostic tests to accurately determine your status.

Diagnosing Leaky Gut Syndrome

To be completely certain, you should consider getting a thorough diagnosis. That's all well and good. But just where to start?

Start by visiting a health care practitioner or doctor you trust and who understands leaky gut syndrome.

The first test you will undergo is a **lactulose-mannitol test** (PolyetheGlycol Test or PEG). Your body can't use or metabolize water-soluble sugar molecules, both mannitol and lactulose. They're absorbed into your bloodstream. They are different in size and weight and the actual rate of absorption varies.

In a healthy digestive process, the cells digest mannitol easily. On the other hand, the lactulose only digests partially. Therefore, the results of this test should indicate a high level of mannitol and a low level of lactulose for a digestive system that isn't obstructed by leaky gut syndrome.

If the opposite happens, low mannitol and high lactulose, it indicates the presence of leaky gut syndrome.

If your test reveals low levels of both of the sugar molecules, this is most likely that you have a problem dealing with absorption.

It's interesting that many individuals who have a high level of lactulose and a low mannitol (that is the probability of leaky gut syndrome), also suffer with Celiac disease (the inability to digest gluten in wheat and other products), Crohn's disease, and ulcerative colitis.

Your preferred test

If you prefer to do the test at home, a home kit is available. Complete instructions are clearly indicated for you to follow and send it off to a pre-pre-designated lab for analysis.

The test is pretty simple and easy. Firstly, collect a urine sample. This provides the lab with a baseline reading. You'll then drink a mannitol-lactulose solution. After waiting for six hours, you'll collect a second urine sample. You send these to the lab designated in your instructions. The results will reveal your levels. You'll also receive information on reading the results properly.

If the test indicates the development of leaky gut syndrome, it's advisable for you to undergo several more tests, some of which look for a few other health conditions as well.

Dysbiosis

One of these tests is called a **comprehensive digestive stool analysis (CDSA)**. This test reveals the bacterial balance (or imbalance) of your digestive tract. In effect, it detects if dysbiosis is present. That is the technical term for the imbalance. In addition, the test reviews the overall state of your digestive health.

There is also another useful function of this test that determines the presence of Candida in your system. You might remember that we discussed the presence of this fungal infection is closely linked to leaky gut syndrome.

If Candida infection is present, your health-care provider will take a culture to determine the amount of growth and to determine a method for treating it.

The CDSA also measures the status of several digestive functions, level of a pancreatic enzyme, the quantity of short-chain fatty acids and the level of butyric acid in your colon.

Don't get intimidated with their seemingly unpronounceable names, the issue really isn't all that complicated.

According to MayoClinc.com, cholecystokinin is a substance that enables the gallbladder to contract. It also triggers the pancreas to produce enzymes, both of which are essential for proper digestion. Butyric acid helps with raising your metabolism, controlling inflammation and helping you manage stress.

Testing for Parasites

The fact is that approximately 1 in 6 individuals carries at least one parasite, according to the Centers for Disease Control. This is probably the highest this figure has ever been.

The presence of parasites has increased dramatically for several reasons. Contaminated water supplies, the increase and ease of international travel, the growth in day care centers with dozens of children being in contact with each other and sharing toys, and living closer to our pets are just a few of the many possible reasons for the burgeoning parasite population.

You may never have realize that there are parasites living in you, but if you listen to your body closely, it's giving you subtle clues. So subtle, that they can be easily ignored or mistaken for signs of other health issues.

From the list below, you'll be able to see what I mean. These are a few of the indicators of the presence of these tiny creatures.

- Stomach pain
- Muscle aches
- Anemia
- Joint pain
- Bloating
- Itching
- Bloody stool
- Gas
- Coughing
- Unexplained weight loss
- Nervousness
- Unexplained fevers
- Pain
- Teeth Grinding
- Weakened Immune system
- Sleep problems
- Rashes

As you can see, there's a wide range of symptoms and they could be attributed to any number of other more common health issues. That's exactly why the presence of parasites is so difficult to detect. Very often, parasites aren't even considered as a cause of any of these symptoms.

Stool Samples

Stool samples are not perfect and sometimes it's not very accurate. Sometimes this test has to be done several times before any definitive diagnosis can be made.

Many parasites don't linger in your lower intestines and won't show up in a random stool sample. Many are instead located farther up along your digestive tract. In these cases, stool testing would reveal a negative result.

You may be given an oral laxative inducing diarrhea, which pushes the parasite along the tract out, so it does show up in your stool if it's present.

Some physicians skip the stool sample and use a rectal swab instead.

But to get the most accurate diagnosis, it's best to go to a lab specializing in parasitology testing.

Anything else I should get tested?

There are a few other tests can be taken to have a completely accurate diagnosis. You should take them if you suspect you might have leaky gut syndrome.

Just identifying the specific foods or chemicals that are aggravating your system can greatly improve your chances of improving your health condition.

There are two testing methods: an elimination diet and a provocation diet. I'll talk more about these 2 methods in a later chapter.

Another Tests

In addition to the tests mentioned, there are also a few blood tests which could be easily performed to help uncover sensitivities. They measure your body's reaction to antibodies. These same tests are also useful for food allergies and sensitivities to environmental issues.

Make sure you get these tests in a lab that tests specifically for IgG or IgG4 antibodies. Some labs also include testing for IgA, IgE, and IgM.

All these tests need to be conducted by your physician. He or she will be able to interpret the results. Beside of the analysis, some labs will forward you a list of recommendations, including suggestions for a diet plan and other literature on the subject.

Your doctor may suggest one final test to measure your liver's ability to eliminate toxins. Many natural health practitioners do this by giving you an aspirin, a caffeine tablet and two acetaminophen tablets.

Accurate diagnosis

As you can see, it is not easy to diagnose this syndrome accurately. But if a correct diagnosis may help relieve a variety of unrelated ailments and get you feeling well again, it's certainly well worth the effort.

The next chapter is perfect for people who might want to start making some of the right changes in their lifestyle and habits immediately. Let's get started!

Rebalancing the Digestive System

Up to this, you've learned about the causes of leaky gut syndrome. You've also discovered that diagnosing the problem with any accuracy isn't an easy task. You've also probably realized that this syndrome may be harming your system than you thought.

Since this topic is hardly talked about, you're also wondering if anything can be done to improve the situation. It is a sneaky disorder and it masquerades as any number of other ailments.

While you're concentrating on treating it as one condition, you realized it keeps getting worse. In this chapter, you're about to learn some of the tips, tricks, and techniques to outwit this sneaky health condition.

The good news is that leaky gut syndrome can be cured. And what's even better, is that you can accomplish it without the use of harsh, potentially dangerous and harmful medications.

You can take control and be responsible for the state of your health. Recovering from this disorder is solely in your hands. I've got plenty of confidence in you, though.

You'll learn how to change your habits and stick with them. But remember this, your digestive system won't heal overnight. It will take time and determination to get well. Let's start your road to recovery right now!

Listen to Your Body

One very important key to getting well is following your individual needs. You might have ignored your body when it was telling you that something is wrong or you didn't know what it was telling you.

Now that you're armed with a lot more information and awareness than before, you have a wider understanding of what your real health issues are. This means you'll be much more attuned to the clues your body is sending you. Listen to them carefully!

Patience. Perseverance. Persistence.

Always keep these words in mind as you go through your road to recovery. And so are the guidelines that are to follow. Before I even talk about the changes in your diet and any nutritional supplements you need to be taking, I'll provide you with a few secrets others have used successfully.

A quick & easy starter's guide

This first step you can make immediately is very simple. It involves chewing your food. Most of us chew not only too fast, but also too hard.

Relax when you eat. Chew carefully.

How many meals have you eaten in a hurry in the morning? I'm sure most of us are guilty of this.

Chewing is the first step to a healthy digestive tract. Chewing your food is necessary because it increases the surface area of the food.

This means that your digestive system doesn't have to work so hard. As you chew, your body produces saliva that holds digestive enzymes that actually initiate the process of digestion on both the carbohydrates and the fats.

Called parotid glands, located under your tongue, they deliver messages to your digestive tract and your brain telling them what to expect.

1st step to your new lifestyle

If you are seriously determined about taking on this syndrome, you will face many changes in your lifestyle...especially your diet.

As you start your journey, there are a few things to keep in mind. The first involves any food allergies you may have. Most people with this health condition have a few. Any food allergies or even food sensitivities (which may be even more difficult to detect than allergies) should not be ignored. Indeed, treating these is a major key to healing!

Avoiding foods you are allergic to is recommended for a minimum of 4-6 months. If you have numerous food allergies, you may want to seriously consider a rotation diet.

The first step you can take is a process called reseeding the gut. This is a term Frank Lipman uses in his book called, Total Renewal: 7 Key Steps to Resilience, Vitality and Long-Term Health.

It is restoring the beneficial bacteria, or sometimes called probiotics, and tissues to your body.

Probiotics, unlike antibiotics which kill the toxic bacteria, actually give your body an abundance of healthy bacteria that keep your system running smoothly and infections and toxins in at bay.

The dark side of Antibiotics

There are many actions that destroys your system's supply of probiotics (live bacteria and yeasts that are good for your health, especially your digestive system), including consuming too much junk food, those nutritionally empty snacks. In addition, healthy bacteria may be destroyed by the use of some medications.

While antibiotics are obviously helpful in killing the infection causing bacteria, in the process they also destroy some of your good bacteria.

The use of hormones and steroids can also destroy your healthy bacteria. Now you can see that your digestive system easily harmed!

Introducing: The elimination diet

Changing your eating habits is one of the most popular ways of restoring balance in your body. Many individuals use versions of what's called the elimination diet to deal with food allergies, and especially food sensitivities, which far too often are the underlying cause of leaky gut syndrome.

The elimination diet is a simple theory, but not so simple execute. Our hectic lifestyle leaves us with limited amount of time to eat. I'm sure you know what it feels like hurrying to eat your breakfast not wanting to be late to get to the office. Far too often, you probably eat fast food, restaurant take out, and easy-to-prepare packaged foods.

In many ways, this way of eating is nothing more than a coping mechanism. Sometimes it's the only way we can make it through the week. How many people do you know work 40+ hours a week and still have to do laundry, commute and most likely have no time to make dinner.

Microwavable "processed food" and fast food are what busy people usually go for these days. And what happens to real cheese?

It's no surprise your digestive system is not happy.

Say good bye to processed foods

As part of an elimination diet, processed food is the first to go. These foods are filled with additives and unnatural colorings.

You're also required to eliminate refined sugar, refined white flour and grains containing gluten. These, too, can play havoc with your digestive system.

I'm not saying that you should never eat any of these foods again, but take a break from them for now. You can slowly add them back into your diet one food at a time. Then you check your body's response.

This method has 2 advantages:

1. By eliminating many of the worst offenders for a minimum of a month, you're allowing your body to rebalance. In that time, you'll be supplying it with many of the nutrients and probiotics to restore a proper bacteria-flora ratio.

2. It provides your body many nutrients that the packaged, processed, and fast foods don't have.

Withdrawal symptoms

I have to warn you, though. Many individuals begin to feel worse before they feel better. Your body has grown dependent on many of those unhealthy foods -- especially refined sugar!

By withholding these foods your body may produce temporary adverse reactions – withdrawal symptoms. But this will pass. Once the withdrawal symptoms disappear, you'll experience all the benefits that are promised through this method.

For some people it may take a moth of abstinence from these offenders to rebalance and rebuild. For some, it may take longer. It may take up to 3 months before any definitive results can be seen.

So what kind of food should you be taking? It really depends on the diet you've chosen, but it's best to concentrate on eating fresh vegetables and fruits as much as possible.

Go light on the beef and red meat. If possible, I recommend organic meats and free range chickens. Not only are these foods healthier for you, but you'll discover that they actually taste than what you've been eating!

I won't go into any details about a specific diet in this chapter, but you can find a sample of a three-phase elimination diet that may give you some idea of how this works sample in the appendix.

Some of you might think it will be very hard to jump into these new diets. And some might feel it's impossible to go "cold turkey" from processed and packaged food.

I would recommend for you to take baby steps to start the process. Once you start doing this, you may decide that you can wean yourself off the salt-laden packaged and frozen foods stuffed with artificial additives. Any step, large or small, will help you go forward in mending your diet will help.

The balance of bacteria

As mentioned earlier, one of the main symptoms of leaky gut syndrome is the predominance of bad bacteria over good flora. By rebalancing what is imbalance, it's a good idea to ask for some advice from your personal physician or a natural health care provider.

He or she can offer any number of natural methods to facilitate this. The most effective of these include using garlic, oil of oregano capsules, grapefruit seed extract, mathake tea, berberine, capryllic acid, pau d'arco, and tanalbit.

If you have any Candida yeast infection, this is a good time to address it. This fungus actually responds well to not only dietary changes, but to treatment with natural substances.

Simple guidelines

There are a few simple guidelines you should follow:

1.   Eat a low-carbohydrate diet

2.   Avoid sugar, alcohol, and vinegar

3.   Include the use of a high-quality probiotic product.
        A probiotic is an organism that can be most easily
        described as the friendly flora in your intestines.
        And a good one contains millions of live bacteria.

Once you've "reinforce" your system, the added flora not
only help to reestablish your balance, but actually stop the
growth of the bad bacteria as well. It will also boost your
immune system.

One characteristic of Candida is that they are persistent in
surviving. You may discover that even after you diligently
treat your Candida infections with probiotics, some yeast is
still stubbornly clinging to you. In order to clear your system
thoroughly, you may have to use one or more alternative
methods to ensure the infection is gone.

Another word of caution: as you treat your fungal infection,
it may worsen. Don't panic.

The Rotation diet

The rotation diet is good for people who are suffering from
multiple food allergies. This method works well in keeping
your food allergies under control. Some people find it easier
than the elimination diet to start. Basically, you eat

biologically related foods on the same day. Then you wait a minimum of four days before you eat them again.

Why is this diet good for you? For starters, it stops the continuation of any development of new food allergies. While there are some foods that are more widely known to trigger an allergic reaction, just about any food, if eaten too often, can prompt an allergy. Especially if you have leaky gut syndrome.

By using this diet, you can actually eat the foods you have a mild or borderline reaction to, while reducing the symptoms. You might want to test drive this method before going full force.

We all know that different people react differently. While the standard rotation diet usually advises a four-day rotation plan, you may find that a longer period is necessary for some foods.

The most common foods which trigger allergies include wheat, corn, citrus fruits, legumes, and cow's milk. The test drive period is a good time for you to see what fits you best.

Discover the benefits of FOS foods

Most people are not getting your daily requirement of FOS foods. What? You don't even know what FOS is or what it does?

You're not alone. Most people are totally unaware of these foods and of FOS in particular.

FOS stands for **fructooligosaccharide**. This is a specialized type of sugar molecule which actually increases the growth of flora – the good and healthy bacteria.

The foods rich in this molecule include:

- Asparagus
- Bananas
- Barley
- Onions
- Fruit
- Leeks
- Jerusalem artichoke
- Garlic
- Burdock
- Chicory
- Wheat
- Soybeans

When you increase your consumption of these foods, you're helping to rebalance your digestive system.

Fruits and vegetables

I'm sure your mother probably had this talk with you already since we were young about the importance of fruits and vegetables in your diet. But this time we're approaching the issue from a slightly different angle.

There are good scientific and research behind this time-honored advice. These foods are richly endowed with substances called antioxidants. Sound familiar? Antioxidants are good in keeping you from developing such conditions as dangerous as heart disease and cancer. Antioxidants also help to boost your immune system.

For people who suffer from leaky gut syndrome, eating foods rich with antioxidants may have even more meaning for them.

To truly appreciate their importance, you need to understand what they do.

Thanks to Antioxidants!

Our cells are damaged from exposure to free radicals on a daily basis. Sometimes you'll hear these referred to as reactive oxygen species, or ROS.

All of us produce these substances naturally as a response to metabolism. But they are also produced in other ways. They grow quickly when you smoke, drink alcohol, exposed to radiation, drugs and rancid oil.

But those aren't the only way they grow. Exposure to the sun also causes an increase their growth rate and subjects your body to stress.

What are free radicals exactly? They are unstable molecules searching for stability. They look and snatch electrons for themselves to be re-stabilize. And they don't care where they get them!

These harmful substances usually target your cell and mitochondrial membranes, as well as your nervous system and enzymes. This is particularly dangerous because enzymes are essential in ensuring healthy cellular function.

What's worse is that they also have the potential to damage your DNA, which is the structure determining the way in which your cells replicate.

While this occurs in everyone, the danger to your intestinal tract is heightened when it is injured and there is the presence of free radicals. At this point, they occur in such vast numbers that your system can't control them.

Some experts believe that one free radical can potentially affect one million cells. The extent of the damage depends on the ability of your body to recognize what's happening to it and the availability of antioxidant nutrients to combat them.

Working together

There are different types of antioxidants. Each specific type have their own individual tasks that complement the others. To be effective, they must work together. Antioxidants are found in many fruits and vegetables, so it's really no surprise that so many health experts recommend these foods.

By now you probably start to understand how your body works in harmony with what you put in your mouth to keep them in tip top shape.

In addition to fruits and vegetables, nuts and seeds are also rich with antioxidants. The truth is that when eaten in their natural state, most foods have antioxidants. But once they are processed by freezing or using them in packaged and processed foods, their effectiveness depleted.

Detox

Some people like to call this "detox". Have ever you heard of it?

Fruit and vegetable cleaning, or detoxification, is highly recommended by many specialists who treat leaky gut syndrome because it's not only an effective method of detoxification, but it's also gentle on your system.

Before we go deeper into cleansing, I would like to inform you that any change in diet -- especially one which relies on a specific genre of foods exclusively -- should be cleared with your personal physician. He or she has a working knowledge of what kind of changes your body can handle.

In short, fruits and vegetable cleanse your system naturally. You eat only fresh fruits and vegetables for seven to ten days. You can also use olive and canola oils as condiments during this time.

Add fresh fruit and vegetable juices after ten days. These are incredibly powerful and concentrated sources of nutrients that are beneficial for your body. Juices also have the advantage of being able to enhance detoxification pathways, according to Elizabeth LIpski, author of the book, Leaky Gut Syndrome.

As in any type of detoxification, you may experience some discomfort in the first few days. Some people report they develop headaches. This symptom could occur for any number of reasons, including sugar or caffeine withdrawal.

But don't panic. This simply means you're experiencing withdrawal symptoms and the cleansing is working. Toxins are being flushed out of your system.

Handling withdrawal symptoms

Drinking water, diluted fruit juices and decaffeinated herbal teas are effective ways to deal with withdrawal symptoms. This quicken the elimination of toxins.

Some people have reported that they a rash or pimples. This is also another indication the cleansing process is working. These symptoms mean that toxins are being eliminated through your skin. You can ease the situation through steam baths, saunas, and even massaging your skin with a loofa or a soft dry brush.

Constipation is also another symptom some people develop. You may take a fiber supplement to help. You might also discover that psyllium seeds or freshly ground flaxseeds help. Start with one teaspoon of either of these in water then drink quickly before it turns into a gel.

Everything mentioned in this chapter are simply basic guidelines to get you started on adjusting your diet to help heal your health condition. It's easy to start with small steps. Taking a step -- no matter how small – is meaningful. If continued and you add steps as you go along, you'll discover a whole new healthy you!

While you're in your diet adjustment period, you may also want to heighten the effect by taking nutritional supplements. They can help add a punch to your other efforts.

Which supplements should you take? In the next chapter I will give you some ideas about the best supplements to get you started.

Rebalancing With Nutritional Supplements

The last chapters have informed you the importance of transforming your diet from artificial to fresh. It's also possible that you've take steps towards rebalancing at this point. Good for you! But, don't stop there. There are other steps you can take to boost these changes.

They come in the form of nutritional and dietary supplements. While the best form of getting your vitamins, minerals, and antioxidants is obviously through whole, fresh foods, the imbalance in your system may demand additional help.

That's where these amazing nutritional boosts come in. They may give you just the right amount of the needed building blocks to help battle an unhealthy condition that's been allowed to sit in your digestive system for too long.

Once you have rebalanced your digestive system, you can reduce your supplement intake or stop them all together. At the very least, that should be your goal.

So without further ado, let's take a look at the variety of supplements you can take. I will provide you with a variety from which to choose. You're bound to find at least one that helps you in curing your leaky gut syndrome.

Glutamine

Glutamine, it is probably the most important amino acid in the maintenance of both the structure and the function of the intestine. It is essential for a healthy metabolism. You can get it naturally by consuming many high-protein foods.

It's the body's "preferred fuel" for the cells which line the mucosa of your small intestine. These particular cells use glutamine directly rather than waiting for the bloodstream to deliver them.

Another important aspect of this amino acid is that it prevents the translocation of bacteria from the gut into the bloodstream -- a vital aspect to healing leaky gut syndrome.

For these reasons, your body needs a generous quantity of glutamine for the repair and maintenance of a healthy small intestinal lining.

Foods rich in glutamine:

- Beans
- Beef

- beats

- Cabbage

- Chicken

- Dairy products

- Fish

How to obtain additional Glutamine

Considering how important glutamine is in the health of those who suffer with leaky gut syndrome, you may want to seriously consider taking a glutamine supplement. You can purchase this in several forms.

First, you want to look for a supplement marked l-glutamine. It comes in either a capsule or as a powder. According to The Environmental Illness Resource (www. ei-resource.org), you need rather large amounts of this supplement in order for it to be effective. The suggested serving for anyone whose symptoms are moderate to severe is between 5 and 20 grams daily.

Vitamin A

Vitamin A is another essential nutrient for a healthy gastrointestinal tract. It triggers the production of protective antibodies known as SigA. This familiar nutrient also aids in the maintenance of your intestinal mucosa. An added benefit is its ability to ease inflammation.

Vitamin A is vastly available in health food stores, vitamin shops, and even grocery stores. But you may want to search for a specific form of this essential health building block. It's called an emulsion. It'll cost a little more, but it's probably the most effective form. It literally coats the intestinal mucosa, working its way to all the most crucial areas. And it can be taken without any fear of adverse side effects in servings of 20,000 to 25,000 IU daily.

Vitamin B complex

If you suffer from leaky gut syndrome, the family of the **B-complex** of vitamins is under attack. This is no surprise; we've said many times, is the blocking of the absorption of many nutrients.

From all of the Vitamin B's, it's B-12 that is especially threatened by this imbalance of bacteria in your small intestines. And for this reason, you may develop -- in addition to your leaky gut problems -- pernicious anemia. Pernicious anemia occurs when your body is lacking in Vitamin B-12, even though it's apparently receiving an adequate supply through dietary sources and supplementation.

A vitamin B-12 deficiency is quite rare. The body stores several years' worth ensuring you stay healthy. But for those with leaky gut, your body can't access the stores and the nutrient is of no use.

I would like to recommend that you might want to ask your doctor to run a simple blood test to see if you have low B-12 before buying the supplement. Your doctor can find the proper way to help you rebuild your system. B-12 is essential in the proper functioning of your nervous system.

Vitamin C's

Vitamin C is long been known as an effective immune booster. Millions of people take it religiously during cold and flu season to prevent the illness.

There are 2 powerful reasons why it's a supplement worth taking if you suffer from this disorder. As mentioned before, leaky gut syndrome is partially caused by the presence of free radicals in your system. Scientists have discovered that antioxidants are the most effective way to neutralize the damaging effects of these scavenger molecules. And vitamin C is a potent antioxidant!

But more than that, the immune-boosting power of this vitamin can help heal this disorder as well.

4,500 mg of vitamin C daily is recommended. Start taking this supplement slowly starting from 500 to 1,000 mg daily and gradually increase the dosage. See how you feel.

Sometimes taking large amounts of vitamin C can backfire and cause digestive issues such as diarrhea.

Vitamin E

Vitamin E probably ranks second only to vitamin C in its usefulness. It's rich in antioxidant that heals tissues from free-radical damage. Like vitamin C, it also possesses incredible immune-boosting powers.

As you embark on your elimination diet, besides eating all the right foods, consider supplementing your diet with this powerful source of healing.

Again, you may want to start off slowly and gradually. Let your body adjust to any new supplement you're introducing. According to the Office of Dietary Supplements, an adult can safely take 1,000 mg a day.

Magnesium

According to scientific research, **magnesium** deserves your attention if you suffer from leaky gut syndrome. It seems that those who suffer from this condition and from one of the consequential disorders it triggers -- fibromyalgia -- appear to be prone to magnesium deficiency.

This deficiency occurs when your intestinal walls become inflamed and they damage many of the carrier proteins necessary for the transportation of this mineral.

This problem stems not only from consumption, but absorption also. You may be suffering from a lack of magnesium, even though you're eating foods that are rich with this mineral. That's why it's vital that the inflammation is treated as quickly as possible.

You can safely take a maximum of 350 mg of magnesium daily.

Zinc

Zinc is a newly well-known healing substance and is perfect specifically for cells with a rapid turnover, just like those of the small intestine mucosa. Being replaced rapidly (approximately every 4 days), these cells require zinc to strengthen the integrity of the intestinal lining.

Recent studies reveal that zinc actually heals leaky gut syndrome. And it may ease or heal Crohn's disease as well.

Even though you might be eating lots of food rich in zinc, it is a good idea to take this mineral supplements. Your body uses zinc at rapid rate, so it may be difficult to keep refilling. It's not surprising that research performed recently by Dr. Keith Eaton, working for an organization called Biolab based in London, uncovered that zinc is the most common nutritional deficiency among leaky gut syndrome sufferers.

Most natural health experts recommend servings between 50 to 80 mg daily. This range is large enough to rebalance any deficiency of zinc. While usually more is better, they also advise not to take more than 100 mg a day.

With this level of supplementation, it helps bolster your immune system. But taking too much will actually have the opposite effect on your immune system.

It is also recommended to take zinc in conjunction with copper because taking zinc supplements can actually deplete your copper level. For every 15 mg of zinc you take, you should take 1 mg of copper.

Make sure you choose your nutritional supplements carefully. You should not only inform your health care provider that you're taking these supplements, but also ask for advice. He or she knows your specific symptoms and has run blood tests that may shed light on what nutrients you're lacking.

The best way to go is to work hand in hand with your physician who understands leaky gut syndrome.

Herbal supplements is another method of supplementing to choose from. Many of these plants are packed with vitamins, minerals and phytonutrients that can enhance your health.

The following chapter lists just a few of the very best herbs for this syndrome.

Rebalancing With Herbs

Rebalancing your body with herbs is an old and honored tradition and potentially an effective way to improve your health. A wide variety of cultures have turned to plants to help them restore health and cure many ailments.

Many of the prescription medications that so many of us depend on today were actually originally taken from plants. Aspirin and some heart medications are only two prime examples.

So it only makes sense that to help heal your leaky gut syndrome, you may want to turn to these amazing nutritional natural aids.

I've said it before, and I will say it again: before you embark on any supplementation program, be sure you consult with your personal physician. Tell her or him what you're planning to take to ensure there are no conflicts with any prescription medications you're taking.

Before deciding on an herbal regimen, consider consulting a professional herbalist. An herbalist has spent years studying herbs through an accredited school. He or she will be able to help you pinpoint exactly what will help your symptoms and condition.

The herbalist may give you a list of suggestions. In the meantime, here are some suggestions to get you thinking about what's possible.

Slippery elm

If you're at all familiar with herbal remedies, then you might already know something about the herb **slippery elm**. For more than 100 years, professional herbalists have relied on this plant as a healing salve for wounds, burns, skin inflammation, boils, ulcers . . . need I go on?

It also happens to be an effective agent when taken internally as well. In addition to its ability to treat coughs, sore throats, and diarrhea, this versatile herb can also help remedy stomach problems.

Slippery elm possesses a mucilage. Mucilage is a substance which turns to gel when mixed with water. It forms a coat and soothes your mouth, throat, stomach, and intestines.

In addition, this amazing herb also contains an abundance of antioxidants. We've already discussed that can help reduce free radicals, which in turn aid in the development of leaky gut. According herbalists, this herb particularly relieves inflammatory infections in the bowel.

It also triggers reflux stimulation of the nerve endings in your gastrointestinal tract, which eventually lead to an increase in mucus secretion. That's a good thing. This increase in production protects your gastrointestinal tract from such disorders as ulcers and acidity.

In essence, slippery elm soothes and calms an inflamed and damaged gut lining. Specifically, it's this soothing action which eventually allows the antioxidants to perform their tasks.

Peppermint tea

Peppermint tea has been used by herbalists to treat a variety of stomach problems and any other number of disorders for a very very long time.

Peppermint tea drink has a calming and numbing effect. It also kills certain kinds of bacteria. Even research is now showing that it is a credible defense against indigestion and irritable bowel syndrome.

The ingredients in this herbal tea calm the stomach and promote the flow of bile, a needed ingredient in the digestion of fats. This enables food to pass through the stomach more quickly.

How to prepare Peppermint tea:

If you have been growing this herb in your garden, use the dried leaves of the plant. Prepare your tea by steeping one teaspoon of the dried leaves in a cup of boiling water for approximately 10 minutes.

Then strain and cool the mixture. For the best results, drink it four or five times a day between meals.

If you are not in to growing your own peppermint, this tea is widely available in the supermarket. You can also purchase enteric-coated capsules. These are specially coated so the capsule may pass through the stomach into the intestine.

1-2 capsules taken at least twice a day is recommended. Some herbalists say the optimum serving is 2 capsules 3 times daily. The latter recommendation is especially pertinent if you have irritable bowel syndrome.

Chamomile tea

Another well-known and greatly used tea that may benefit you is **chamomile tea**. This tea is already considered a calming and relaxing agent; many individuals drink it as part of their nightly bedtime ritual.

In addition, this tea is filled with strong antispasmodic and anti-inflammatory ingredients, which can be effective in the treatment of stomach problems and intestinal cramps.

It's a recommended remedy for the cramping and pain of the bowels associated with irritable bowel syndrome. Additionally, chamomile tea helps with the excessive gas and bloating of the intestines.

All you need is a single cup of chamomile tea daily. That's certainly easy enough!

This tea can be purchased practically anywhere. It's not only available in health food stores and vitamin shops, but it can be found commercially in just about any grocery store.

Marshmallow root

It's an herb? Yes, it is. While the herb **marshmallow root** has nothing to do with that yummy campfire treat s'mores, it has everything to do with soothing the irritated mucous membranes of your upper respiratory tract and your digestive tract. Perfect for healing leaky gut syndrome.

Don't let the name fool you. Marshmallow root -- many times referred to as mallow -- has a healing history that literally extends thousands of years in the past. This root is extremely effective in helping almost all problems related to the inflammation of your digestive tract.

This supplement is not as easy to find. But you should have no trouble finding it at health food stores and vitamin shops. And of course, if you can't find it any place else, you can always purchase it online.

Herbs that eliminate Parasites

The presence of parasites in many individuals who suffer from leaky gut syndrome was mentioned earlier. There is a combination of three herbal tinctures you may want to take that can help you rid your body of the parasites.

One of the biggest advantages of this healing blend is its effectiveness on more than 100 different types of parasites. With the proper serving, it kills not only the adult parasites but also the eggs as well. The tinctures are black walnut green, wormwood, and cloves.

When I talk about the black walnut green tincture, I'm referring to the use of the green hull that surrounds the nut of the black walnut tree. According to many herbalists, its ability to kill parasites is near miraculous. It's important that the hull is used while it is green. Once it turns black, it loses its active ingredients.

In many instances, the black walnut supplements found in vitamin shops and health food stores are made with the hull after it has turned black. You may want to work closely with a professional licensed herbalist in order to ensure your black walnut tincture is effective.

The walnut and wormwood are the herbs that effectively kill off the adult parasites, while the third herb, the cloves tincture, kills the eggs.

Echinacea

Echinacea is one of the most widely used herbs in this country, and with good reason. Its history goes back at least 400 years. Native Americans used it to treat infections and wounds. In fact, you'll discover that this amazingly versatile herb is probably the closest you'll find to an "all-purpose" herb. Uses include treating scarlet fever, malaria, blood poisoning, and even diphtheria.

Echinacea probably reached its peak in popularity in the 18th and 19th centuries in The United States. With the rise of prescription antibiotics, it quickly faded from the public. But now it's making a stunning comeback as people discover the dangers of using harsh medications.

It is not surprising that it is gaining in popularity since research confirms its effectiveness. Several studies reveal that its active ingredients improve the immune system, reduce inflammation, and possesses antioxidant qualities.

For many herbalists, Echinacea is the first choice in the treatment of Candida as well as several other infections.

Many individuals find using Echinacea, the well-established herb that's a natural antibiotic, helps them in avoiding the overuse of prescription antibiotics. Instead of visiting their doctor and filling a prescription, they reach for this herb.

Of course, this herb won't work for all infections, but it helps those who tend to overuse or even abuse antibiotic medications.

Taking Echinacea

Most herbalists suggest that you take Echinacea 3 times daily for seven to 10 days in order to ensure that you receive its full antibiotic benefits.

There are a number of forms for you to choose from. If you're lucky enough to have some fresh herbs, you'll want to dry the root or the plant itself and use it as a tea. For this purpose, you'll need 1 to 2 grams.

If you're using a standardized tincture extract, you'll need 2 to 3 ml of the liquid. As a powdered extract, you'll need 300 mg of the standardized powder.

Goldenseal

Goldenseal is another favorite of herbalists in the treatment of leaky gut. It is an herb that, like Echinacea has a legendary reputation when it comes to digestive issues.

This herb has just the right combination capacity that can make it an invaluable dietary supplement if you're troubled with a leaky gut. It works fast on digestive tissues and it's a natural antibiotic too.

Many herbalists will pair this herb with Echinacea to create a powerful supplement that not only helps the digestive tract, but improves your immune system also.

Goldenseal widely available — you can find it in health food stores, vitamin shops, and even grocery stores. You have your choice in taking the tablet form or the capsule variety.

Pau d'arco

This might be something you've never heard of before. Pau d'arco, a plant native to South America, has been widely used to control pain, keep arthritis at bay, and to treat inflammation.

Pau d'arco is often used to treat Candida infections and any number of bacterial infections. You're already well aware that Candida is a disorder that goes hand-in-hand with leaky gut. This herb also attacks another symptom of leaky gut -- the presence of parasites.

You have a few choices in the form you take it. A few examples will be in tablet form, dried bark teas and tinctures. You can find any of these at health food and vitamin shops. You may also want to request a tailor-made formula that fits your unique needs from a professional herbalist.

The most common serving is 300 to 500 mg in capsule form three times a day. If you're using a tincture, you'll use between ½ to I ml two to three times daily.

So far we've covered many of the ways to rebalance your body through diet and supplementation -- both nutritional and herbal.

Ok, we've covered a lot...but what about that other cause and aggravator of leaky gut syndrome: stress? Everyone of us experience it. At work, at home, at school, even in your daily commute. Is there anything that can be done to eliminate that?

The answer is NO. There is no way any of us can eliminate stress from our body. The good news is that you can learn how to manage it intelligently. The following chapter gives you some clues on how to do just that!

Stress Management and Beyond

Stress. We hate it, but we all have it. It certainly is one of the ongoing problems of the 21st century. Today, you're probably feeling the stress more than ever. Stress has become an unspoken but omnipresent fact of life.

Believe it or not, stress has become the highest cause of ill health. Did you know that the World Health Organization has listed on-the-job stress as one of the top ten reasons for poor health? In fact, one in three adults suffer from moderate to extreme stress. That's 1/3 third of the U.S. population!

No one can go about their day without experiencing some type stress. It can be work-induced, or caused by the concern of payment of bills or a super-tight schedule. Stress is unavoidable.

Stress can be a good thing...in moderation. It can be motivating. It'll push us to work harder for us to achieve our goals we might not have accomplished otherwise. And there are those individuals who say they work best under stress.

It certainly served our ancestors well. The caveman experienced stress when confronted with dangers such as the presence of a woolly mammoth. Once the stress mechanism kicked in, it gave our prehistoric ancestor the strength and energy either to fight the large creature or to run from it.

But in prehistoric times, our ancient ancestors didn't deal with stress on a daily or even hourly basis, as we do today. They encountered stress far less often. The caveman's reaction to stress actually was a life-saving mechanism instead of the health-draining reaction it has become.

Reacting to Stress

We deal with tense situations at work, at home, and basically anywhere we go to. Our reactions to stressful situations are reflected in our physical well-being. That's right -- your reaction to the pressures of daily life has a direct bearing on your physical body.

As a matter of fact, how we choose to react to stress affects the status of our health. For starters, it's well known that prolonged exposure to pressures can actually lower your immune system!

If you allow stress take over, can take a devastating toll on your body. Not only you will look old and tired, but it will affect your body internally. Your reaction to stress may be one of the causes of leaky gut syndrome.

The truth is, we can't avoid stress. No matter how hard we try to avoid it, it's a part of our lives. This means you have to learn how to live with it. And I'm not talking about just giving in to the tension. I'm speaking about how to meet it and beat it and keep your cool -- and your health.

The good news is that studies reveal that taking specific steps, like beginning certain programs, actually produce physical and chemical changes in your body that help you to feel better.

Let's start your stress-reduction program

Knowing that controlling your stress can improve your leaky gut syndrome, you would want to start as soon as possible. But first, you need to do a thorough examination of your life to see if stress is affecting you.

Is that necessary? Yes, it does...trust me. There are symptoms that can clue you in to this, but you have to be able to recognize them. It's possible that you're experiencing them but not realizing the cause. Leaky gut syndrome is a perfect example. Even if you treat it nutritionally, you may find it recurs if stress is clogging your life.

Watch for the signs

Everyone's reaction to stress is different. It differs from how your spouse may react or from your friend's. How you react is a very personal, very individualized response. The physical symptoms you develop may not be the same as everyone else's.

Even though it might not be noticeable at first, but I guarantee that there is a set of signs that indicate the situation is affecting your body. I've listed some of them below.

* *Pay attention to your feelings.* Are you feeling anxious, irritable, fearful? Are you experiencing mood swings you don't understand? Even feeling unexplained embarrassment can all be attributed to an emotional response to stress.

- *Carefully review what you're thinking.* When you're "stressed-out," it's reflected in your thoughts. You may find you're more critical of yourself, or you may have noticed that you have a shorter concentration span.

- *Are being more forgetful than usual?* Are you having trouble making decisions? Other signs that stress may be harming you physically (and mentally) include a preoccupation with the future, repeating the same thoughts over and over, and the constant fear of failure.

- *Study your behavior.* If you're coping to stress, it surely will reveal itself in your behavior. Do you find yourself crying for no apparent reason, or over small trivial things?

Are you suddenly short-tempered with friends or family members? This is usually one of the first signs that you're not handling stress very well.

- *Watch if there's a change in your eating habit.* Have you noticed a change in your normal eating habits -- either eating more or suddenly having no appetite?

- Other than food, some individuals deal with stress by turning to alcohol. Has there been a change in the amount you drink in a day? You may also find you're taking up cigarette smoking again, or if you've never quit, you're smoking more than usual.

There are other signs such as nervous laughter or teeth grinding or jaw clenching. Other people find that they are more accident prone when stress is adversely affecting them.

Let's look at some other physical symptoms of a stressed out body. We already know that stress can eventually cause or worsen leaky gut syndrome. But there are many other signals:

- Sleep problems
- Tight muscles
- Headaches
- Unexplained fatigue
- Cold or sweaty hands
- Neck or back problems
- Stomach distress
- Rapid breathing
- Pounding of the heart
- Dry mouth

And this list only touches the tip of the iceberg. But even from this, you can see how integrated your emotional and physical health is.

Now that you know it's virtually impossible to avoid stress, you then need to learn how to deal with stress intelligently. You may not know where to begin. Start with small simple steps and I guarantee you'll eventually feel it in a big way.

There are long-term solutions, but firstly, here are few steps you can take immediately to help lower your stress level.

Long deep breaths

Sounds too simple? But it is that simple. You just have to remind yourself to do this (most people forget!). When you are stung by stress, one of the first physical signs is shallow breathing. Ironically, this response only creates more stress!

Pay attention to your breathing and call a quick time out to do a review of your body. Scan your body for any possible physical tension. In addition to that shallow breathing, do you have a tight chest? Some individuals actually hold their breath without even knowing it.

Shallow breathing results from a decreased supply of oxygen in your bloodstream and that leads to muscle tension. But that's only the beginning. Next you will experience a headache. At the very least, you begin to feel even more anxious.

Instead of allowing this chain to continue, realize what's going on and stop! It will take some practice. Take a minute -- yes, I mean 60 seconds -- to slow down and breathe deeply.

Inhale deeply through your nose and exhale through your mouth. Inhale enough breath that your lower abdomen rises and falls. Exhale slowly as you count to 10.

In the beginning you might think that it's not working. But this is a wonderful technique, and it's a technique you must learn how to do. Practice it. You'll see how effective it can be.

Practice time management

How you go through your day can also create stress. Do you spend most of your day running from appointment to appointment, eating in a hurry on the run? And just to get home to do more rushing only with different destinations and purposes?

Over-committing or over-booking your day is one of the major causes of stress. You might say, "I have too many things to do and too little time!" Instead of throwing up your hands, explaining "That's just how life is," try to manage your time.

And yes, I know that it won't be easy. As a matter of fact, it may take you several attempts to master this. You may have to make some adjustments or even eliminate one or two items from your schedule sometimes. You must prioritize your tasks. Aren't the small adjustments worth your good health?

Plan ahead. I know it's easier than said, but it can be done. Start by making a reasonable schedule for the day ahead. Include in this schedule time for stress-reduction exercises as well.

Many people like to try do all their needs at once. Multitasking is a good thing, but this usually results in nothing getting accomplished. You only end up frustrated because another day has passed. You feel -- and perhaps rightly so -- as if you've accomplished nothing important.

Even though they stress us out, yet many of us continue to function this way. It's time to try a different approach. Make a list (yes, I know you've done this before, but bear with me) of all the tasks that face you for that day.

Take it one task at a time

Take it one task at a time. Let me repeat that. Only tackle one job at a time. Once it's done, check it off your list. Then and only then allow yourself to do the next task on your list.

Prioritize. List the tasks according to their importance. List and tackle the most important activities first. Don't procrastinate. We all have different reasons for putting certain tasks off. We either dread performing them, or we dread who we have to interact with. Push all those fears aside and just get it over with!

As a matter of fact, most efficient people get the hardest tasks first or as soon as possible. By doing so, they actually get them done and don't have time to . . . stress about it! And, most importantly, the tasks are done and over with and won't linger on to the next day.

The key to be able to manage time properly is not to over schedule yourself or overburden yourself with tasks that are impossible to finish. You may be tempted to schedule meetings back to back with little if any time in between. Don't do that. Estimate time wisely for events and meetings. That way you're not running behind, stressed because you're late for the next event.

Don't isolate yourself. Sometimes you need some time alone to accomplish some tasks. But, I don't spend all my time alone. That's not healthy.

Seek out others. After some time, you need to take a break from what you are doing. I know that sometimes you feel you can't even take a toilet break because you're on a deadline. But even when working against this type of stress, you need to take an occasional break.

Walk to the coffee room to talk to someone. Visit your colleague at his or her desk. Heck, just go down the hall to talk with the receptionist. But keep in touch with others.

Many freelancers working from home take a day or several hours to work at a different location other than their home such as a coffee shop or library. This is a healthy habit. It keeps them connected with others. And a change in scenery is not a bad thing.

Talk!

This suggestion is a goes hand in hand with the last one. One of the reasons for stress is the inability to talk to anyone about your work . . . your concerns . . . your problems. Even talking about your puppy helps to relieve stress.

If you're a little shy to talk to other people, try writing your concerns out. Just putting your problems or your decisions on paper can lay them out in such a way that an answer pops into your head. A diary at hand will be good.

Laugh!

"Laughter is the best medicine." If it's not the best medicine, it certainly ranks high up there with the top two or three!

No matter what happens try don't lose your sense of humor. Learn how not to take yourself too seriously. And above all, learn how to laugh at yourself.

The one-minute vacation

Take a moment to close your eyes. Imagine a place where you feel relaxed and happy. Then take note of all the details of this place. Imagine not only the physical attributes (is it a beach?) but try to imagine smells, feel the temperature, listen for the sounds that would be here.

This isn't just to see how creative your imagination is. Research now shows that visualizing a tranquil scene can actually lift you from your stressful situation.

Can't do this on your own? You may want to purchase a CD of guided imagery exercises. You can also find plenty on YouTube for free!

Are you comfortable?

Again, this isn't a rhetorical question. What you are wearing can actually contribute to your stress. In order to keep stress at bay, dress as comfortably as you can within the dress code of your workplace.

But don't constrict yourself unnecessarily. If you're female and have to wear dress shoes, you may want to choose flat ones instead of heels.

Beyond what you wear, make sure your chair and table are comfortable and that the temperature is within a certain comfortable range. This might be a problem when you're in an office where your employer provides everyone the same set of furniture. If this becomes a problem, try requesting a more suitable chair or table for yourself.

The same goes with air conditioning. Sometimes it is from an internal general machine for the whole building/floor. Make sure to bring a jacket if your office is too cold. Don't wait until your environment becomes intolerable to make changes! Being physically comfortable reduces your stress more than you think.

Know your limits

Knowing your limits doesn't mean you're weak. Everyone has a limit. Recognize what you can and can't do. Some people waste their time in a vain attempt to control events or – even worse -- other people in order to accomplish their goals. This never works.

Steven Covey said it best in his 7 Habits of Highly Effective People when he told us to know what we can and can't change. Then focus on those items we have control over!

When you're faced with a stressful situation, ask yourself this question first: "Is this really my problem?" It you answer no, then walk away from it.

If the answer is yes, firstly identify any steps you can take immediately to remedy it. And once you have handled it satisfactorily, set it aside and be confident in your actions. Don't try to second guess yourself.

Compromise

Many people get upset and stressed out when someone acts other they believe they should. You can avoid unwanted stress by learning how to compromise. Some get upset when people don't see eye to eye. Compromise. It's much less stressful than confrontation, and it goes a long way to reducing your stress.

You can use these steps right away starting right now. Next, I have some activities you can begin today -- or in the near future.

Yoga

Yoga's popularity has increased in the Western and more and more people consider yoga as a stress busting activity. In fact, yoga is a practice that dates back at least 5,000 years. It is, without a doubt, the oldest form of self-development.

Some employers actually offer yoga to their employees. These employers know that happy and healthy workers are more productive and creative. Instead of dealing with their stress, these employees are busy dealing with the details of their jobs.

Yoga is an ancient practice that includes controlled breathing and meditation, mental imagery, and stretching and physical movement.

Interestingly, the word yoga comes from the same root as the word yoke. And this isn't just a coincidence. Yoke, of course, means to bring together. Yoga, in a very real way, does just that. It brings together the mind, body, and spirit.

Many individuals use yoga as a method of transformation, but more than that, its popularity can be attributed to its effectiveness in stress management and improving your physical health.

What exactly can yoga do?

You'd be surprised at what other benefits yoga can bring you. A few of yoga's advantages include:

- Reduction of stress
- Improved sleeping habits
- Reduction of cortisol levels
- Allergy symptom relief
- Asthma symptom relief
- Decrease in blood pressure

- Slower heart rate

- Reduction in anxiety

- Reduction in muscle tension

- Increased strength

- Improved flexibility

- Slowing of the aging process

Before you start fearing that you have to do difficult poses, let me inform you that there are many of which aren't of the pretzel-bending sort. And this is especially true as a beginner. The moves are simple yet highly effective in relieving stress.

Basically, yoga is all about controlled breathing and stretching of the body into a variety of poses. Ironically, your body not only realizes a natural state of relaxation, but it's also energized at the same time.

The benefits of yoga aren't just all in your head. Recent research confirms that your physical body also undergoes a transformation. As you practice yoga, your body releases high levels of a chemical called serotonin, a substance that induces feelings of well-being. You will be more flexible and gain long lean muscles.

As you start looking for a yoga class, you'll discover that there are many different types of yoga. Some practices have goals that target spiritual transformation, some for losing weight, and others simply aim to help you reduce stress. Make sure you ask what type of yoga the class involves and the ultimate aim of it before enrolling.

If you're searching specifically for a style that reduces your stress without any spiritual implications, you're probably looking for a Hatha yoga class.

You can do a research on yoga classes near you and there are many DVDs and books available that will show you the various poses as well. If you are on a budget, you can start by watching some videos on YouTube. But it is recommended to consult a professional. There are also yoga teachers that can teach you at the comfort of your own home.

Meditation

Another form of relaxation is meditation. It's no surprise that meditation is rooted in the practice of yoga. You don't need to learn yoga to meditate. Meditation is a powerful relaxation tool. Not only that, this simple practice can bring about positive health changes in your body!

Thankfully, you don't need to be a Yogi to mediate. A Yogi is a member of such eastern religions as Buddhism, Hinduism, and Taoism who practices the ancient art of meditation.

I have to warn you though, meditation won't be easy and can be frustrating for first timers. But the benefits outweigh the frustration.

It's true that thousands of years ago, meditation was once confined to the realms of the spiritual elite. And no, to reap the real benefits of mediation, you don't need to subscribe to any religion or even have any desire to seek a spiritual plateau.

Typically, the word meditation conjures up an image of a Buddhist monk in a cave contemplating the meaning of life. One of the best known of these monks is Milarepa, who spent years isolated in a cave in the mountains of Tibet seeking enlightenment.

Meditation: simple and inexpensive

Meditation is simple to perform and inexpensive. It doesn't require any special equipment, although some individuals invest in soothing music and aroma therapy essential oils to help them slip into the meditative state. They are not necessary, though.

If you're still hesitant because you're intimidated by the thought of contorting your legs pretzel-like into the classic, but uncomfortable-look full lotus position, don't worry. You don't.

As a matter of fact, you can meditate anywhere in any position. There are walking meditations. In fact there's a practice of this art that you perform while you walk through a large labyrinth. You can meditate while you're riding the subway, in a waiting room, or even in the midst of a business meeting. (Just be sure you're not the person giving the presentation. Awkward!)

Meditation is not a magic trick

Many people still have the impression that meditation is some hocus-pocus magic trick. It isn't. It is for clearing your mind and relaxation. It is now becoming more and more of an acknowledged mind-body complementary medicine, recognized even by allopathic physicians.

Complementary medicine is any useful aid you perform in addition to conventional medicine. For you, as a sufferer of leaky gut syndrome, it doesn't mean you abandon your elimination diet or your other treatments. It merely means that you meditate along with every other therapy.

Meditation works for stress-reduction because it takes your physical body into a heightened state of relaxation and it calms your mind. The goal is to eliminate the jumble of thoughts from your mind. When you can reach this state you'll be utterly impressed with just how good you feel!

What's great about meditation is that its marvelous relaxing effect doesn't end when you've completed your meditation session. A session, which is usually 15-20 minutes, can help you tackle the rest of day no matter what's thrown at you!

Mayoclinic.com says it best. It calls the effects of meditation as "clearing away the information overload that builds up every day and contributes to your stress." How often are you preoccupied with what happened in the past and the "what ifs" of the future. Meditation puts you squarely in the present – where you should be and enjoy.

The emotional benefits of this ancient practice include:

- **Decreasing negative emotions**
- **Viewing your stressful situations from a different perspective**
- **Increasing an awareness of yourself**
- **Learning to focus on the present moment**

- Creating a clear stress-management program

That's really only a small -- but vital -- part of the power of meditation.

It also have been revealed by modern research that this practice can actually improve certain medical disorders. In addition to helping you with your leaky gut syndrome, it has been known to help a wide array of health problems, including:

- Sleep issues
- Drug abuse
- Alcohol abuse
- Allergies
- Anxiety
- Asthma
- Pain
- Binge eating
- High blood pressure
- Cancer
- Depression
- Fatigue
- Heart disease

From a research at Harvard University, it estimates that stress accounts for 50 % - 90 % of all doctor's visits. Wow! Who would have thought it?

Most of our stress is related to work. The following statistics are really quite eye-opening.

Stress is cited for nearly 20 % of all the absenteeism in the workplace. It's the cause of nearly 40 % of companies' turnover rate in employees.

And that's not all, but stress is also responsible for approximately 60 % of all workplace accidents and nearly 30 % of both short- and long-term disabilities.

As you can see, you're not alone if you're feeling the modern-day pressures of stress.

How meditation can help

It sounds easy right? Just sit quietly, calm your mind, and help to heal your body. As I've mentioned before, meditation can take great practice to master, but the healing process is really can be that easy. Research is uncovering some surprising results.

High blood pressure is the first health conditions that modern research realized can be helped through meditative practices. It's especially useful to people who have moderately high blood pressure. This finding has been proven over and over again during the last quarter century. For some people, their blood pressure has improved; reduced by 25 mmHg or more.

In another clinical study, those individuals with chronic pain exhibited a reduction of nearly 50 % in their symptoms through meditation. This reduction lasted for some up to 4 years following the initial meditation training.

There are thousands of other studies on the medical benefits of meditation. Far too many to put them all here. But you get the idea.

Choosing your form of meditation

There are different types of meditation? Yes, there are. That's one of the beauties of this practice. You can choose the type that meets your needs wherever you may be -- and whatever level you're at.

Guided meditation is one of the most popular ways to meditate. It is also called guided imagery or visualization. With this form, you create mental images of places or specific situations that you find relaxing and soothing.

To get the most of this, use as many senses as possible. Imagine not only the visual setting, but also fill in as many details as you can, like what you smell and what you feel through your touch. Recreate the sounds of your scene — wave crashing, birds chirping. Even try to feel the textures of your location -- the sand between your toes, the feel of walking barefoot. You can it a step further to what you taste in your imagination.

Many people like to start with a guide or a specific teacher when they use this technique. And that may be how you want to start. Or you may want to buy a CD that guides you. There are some very good methods. And again, you can also find plenty online for free such as YouTube.

Mantra meditation

Other people meditate with the aid of what's called a mantra. In this method, you silently repeat a calming word or phrase to help you focus. The word can be as simple as love or peace. Or if you're more spiritual, you may want to repeat a word or phrase you find as part of your religious practice. Many use "shalom."

Then there's mindfulness meditation. It's really all about increasing your awareness and your acceptance of living in the moment.

In this form of meditation, you focus your attention on what you experience during your meditation session such as noticing the rhythm of your breathing. Or instead of clearing your mind of thoughts, you observe your thoughts and emotions without passing judgment on them.

The other 2 meditations incorporates physical movement. The first is Qi gong. In addition to meditation and physical movement, it also involves performing breathing exercises.

Qi gong is an ancient Chinese healing and energy tradition. The aim of these exercises -- both the physical and the breathing -- is to "cleanse, strengthen, and circulate the life energy." In Chinese, your life energy is called Qi or Chi.

According to proponents, this practice not only leads to better health and vitality, but it also produces a tranquil mindset. Just as with other forms of meditation, research shows that Qi gong can help a wide variety of health problems. These include asthma, fibromyalgia, arthritis, headaches, pain, cancer, chronic fatigue, cardiovascular disease, and even cancer.

Step into meditation

You can start practicing meditation right now. There are basic simple steps for you to follow. As you progress farther into this practice, you may want to take a class in order to meditate with others. Or you may decide to buy a book on the topic to learn more about it. But for now, I'll give you a taste of how this simple relaxation method is about.

Your location. You need to seek out a quiet and comfortable place where you won't be disturbed. This means no television in the background and turn off the sound of your mobile phone as well. If you want music, use some that is recommended for this practice. It will relax you without interrupting you. You can also use essential oils to relax you even more.

Good posture. About all practitioners agree: mediate with a straight back. Some individuals lie down during their meditation. There aren't actually many rules in this practice, but be aware that you're much more likely to fall asleep when you're in a lying position than to actually have a meditative session -- especially when you're still new to it.

Center yourself. It's difficult to meditate right after work or any other activities that requires a lot of thinking. Quiet yourself first. Give yourself time to unwind and relax from anything in your day that is pressing on your mind. You'll find that it's a lot easier to meditate after doing so.

Concentrate on your breathing. How we breathe actually affects our mind. One major key to an effective meditation is to concentrate on your breathing.

You need to be fully conscious of your breathing. Many individuals imagine they're breathing in peace as they inhale.

As you concentrate on your breathing, try to put any other thoughts aside. Once in a while your thoughts will crop up in your thinking. Be aware of it and gently whisk it away. Continue to concentrate on your breath.

Calming the mind

The last and hardest step is calming the mind completely. Most likely it won't happen on your first attempt. This will not happen overnight. You will find your mind wandering and thoughts will start to distract you. This is normal. Don't react or get upset. Just keep gently pushing them away. Eventually, with enough sessions, clearing your mind will become easier.

Don't worry and think that just because you can't clear your mind completely in the beginning that you will not receive any healing benefits. Because you are.

You are one step closer to learning the ancient healing art of meditation. You'll be amazed how quickly this can change your mood and perspective. You'll also be pleased as you notice the stresses of the day are less apt to zap your energy.

Exercise

Oh no! Most people don't like to hear that word. Most people would say they don't like to exercise or don't have the time. In some ways, that's understandable. After you come home from work, mentally and physically drained, you really just want to sit down and kick your feet up. Been there, done that.

A lot of people feel like that, but remember you are doing what's best for you. In reality, we'd all feel much better if we would do some physical activity.

As a matter of fact, performing physical activity helps to relieve the stress that normally burdens you by the end of the day.

Exercise doesn't just relieve stress, but it also improves your health. But then, you already knew that! What you might not have realized is that better health can help you get through your day. It's nothing but a win-win situation.

Here's one benefit you'd love to have: endorphins. Exercise boosts the production of endorphins. These are neurotransmitters in your brain, which make you feel good in the simplest terms.

Have you ever heard the term runner's high? It's really the "high" feeling a person gets when more endorphins are in your system. But the beauty of this is that you don't need to run to experience it. Any prolonged physical activity will give you the same feeling!

Not only that, but exercising will improve your mood. Feeling down? Take a 30-minute exercise, even something as simple as a walk. You don't even have to take a vigorous walk to experience a better mood. The next time you come home from work give it a try. You may be surprised at the result!

Are you experiencing trouble sleeping at night? You toss and turn, but somehow you just can't fall asleep. Does your mind refuse to shut off, running through the day's events and even tomorrow's? Try some exercise and you'll say good bye to those sleepless nights.

As you're sleeping better, you'll discover you feel less stress. And it can give you a renewed command over your body -- and your life!

Let's get started!

I've said it before, and I'll say it again. Before you start any exercise program -- even a simple walking regimen -- consult your doctor. This is especially true if you have diabetes. Once you've this, you're ready to begin your new life!

Start gradually. Don't start out at full speed. You may be tempted to jump into an exercise program quickly and thoroughly. It's best, though, to start slowly. And you know this.

Start small and simple, especially if you're not used to regular exercising. Even physical activity at a low level is better than none. And you'll feel better even with only a little movement if your body isn't accustomed to it -- guaranteed! You just have to get off your couch and move!

To start with, your goal is 30 minutes a day. If you're out of shape, you may have trouble doing even this much. Don't give up. Build up to this. With just a little determination and discipline, you'll be able to work your way up to a half hour...then to an hour!

Choose an activity you like. Exercise is exercise. You want to be healthy, but you have to enjoy it too. So don't think you're stuck performing some activity that doesn't suit your lifestyle and your preferences. Heck, even time spent in the garden lovingly tending to your plants can be exercise enough to de-stress you.

Once you've started on your program, make it a habit. This means you make an appointment with yourself and you don't break it. If your employer said he wanted to meet with you Monday at 3 p.m., you wouldn't blow it off, would you? Then don't blow off your daily appointment with exercise!

I know what you might be thinking right now..."it's easier said than done!" Perhaps at the beginning you may think that. But, once you get started, you'll want that feel-good-all-over effect that physical activity brings. Eventually (and this may be difficult to believe), your body will tell you it needs the activity and you'll be looking forward to exercise!

If you have trouble starting and sustaining a program, consider enlisting the help of a good friend or if your wallet allows, hire a personal trainer. Set aside time for the two of you to walk with each other. It might be easier to keep your appointment if you know somebody is sitting on a park bench waiting for you!

And you may just discover that when you exercise with a friend, you're more motivated, more committed and more fun!

After a while, some people start to get bored of the same activity. It's a good idea to have other activities/exercises you like to do as an alternative. Maybe you can alternate between walking and swimming during the week. Give it some thought if you think you're getting bored. Improvise and get creative!

Now that you've got a plan and are ready to start your de-stressing program through physical activity, let's get started and give it a try! You'll discover a whole new wonderful relaxing world ahead of you.

And the beauty of it all, you'll notice that the symptoms associated with your leaky gut syndrome are dramatically reduced!

Conclusion

We are getting close to the end of our journey learning about leaky gut syndrome. You've learned that it's actually nothing less than a stealth disorder, masquerading as any number of other disorders. You've also learned that diagnosing this disorder can be difficult because of the sneakiness of this syndrome.

If you suffer from this disorder, you've also discovered that there is hope at the end of the tunnel. Perhaps you've visited many different doctors and specialists that weren't able to discover a cause to your problems.

You're following all of your doctor's orders, taking the latest and greatest medications, but yet nothing helps. You still suffer with pain.

Is it possible that you actually treated the underlying -- the real -- cause of your health condition? Maybe now you can find some relief!

Treat leaky gut syndrome naturally

Congratulations! Now that you have more information and armed with more knowledge, you now can cure leaky gut syndrome naturally, without the need of harsh prescription drugs.

You are not equipped with the necessary tools to embark on a healing program. You are now ready to start your journey back to robust, good health.

Make the first step to recovery...start with these suggestions and continue working at it, there's nothing that can stop you in curing your leaky gut syndrome!

Bonus:

A Sample Leaky Gut Syndrome Elimination Diet

Phase 1

Remember the elimination diet mentioned before? Here is a sample elimination diet. I'm giving this to you to give you some guidelines to knowing what many diets insist you eliminate from your eating habits in order to ease the symptoms of leaky gut syndrome.

You don't have to follow it to a T. You can easily choose the foods that give you the most trouble on the list and start with that. Any steps you take to toward eating healthier are an excellent start.

The list below consists of foods that you should stop eating for one month to allow your body to begin to heal. These foods are commonly the most troublesome for many people with leaky gut syndrome

- Beans
- Bread
- Caffeine
- Chocolate
- Citrus fruits
- Corn
- Dairy products
- Eggs
- Flour
- Bananas
- Gluten grains (wheat, spelt, kamut, rye, barley)
- Honey
- Kiwi
- Millet
- Mushroom
- Nightshade vegetables (eggplant, peppers, potatoes, tomatoes)
- Oats
- Papaya
- Peanuts
- Pineapple
- Soy products

- Strawberries
- Vanilla extract
- Vinegar
- Yeast

The list below consists of foods you may eat. Choose the foods you like so the diet doesn't get boring or too restrictive for your tastes. You can do the elimination diet and not really miss the foods you can't eat at all!

Stay with this list for a month. Your body will begin to adjust and then you can begin -- slowly -- to add other foods one at a time to your diet.

- Amaranth
- Apples
- Apricots
- Avocados
- Beets
- Berries (except strawberries)
- Bok choy
- Brussels Sprouts
- Carrots

- Cherries
- Cilantro
- Coconut milk
- Dandelion Greens
- Figs
- Grapes
- Kale
- Lettuce
- Nectarines
- Olive oil
- Onions
- Parsnips
- Peaches
- Pears
- Pine nuts
- Plums
- Pumpkin seeds
- Quinoa
- Rice, brown and wild
- Spinach
- Sprouts
- Sunflower seeds

Phase 2

Gradually add the following foods below to the "allowed" list. Add one food at a time and wait three days before you add another one to see how your body reacts. If the food gives you an allergic reaction or your body doesn't react well to it, then stay away from it for another month.

- Bananas
- Beans
- Papaya
- Chicken
- Fish
- Nightshade vegetables
- Pineapple
- Soy
- Turkey

Phase 3

Again, gradually add the following foods one at a time in three-day increments. If you get an adverse reaction, then eliminate the food for another month.

- Alcohol
- Caffeine
- Chocolate
- Oranges
- Kiwi
- Peanuts
- Sesame seeds
- Strawberries
- Refined sugar
- Pea

Phase 4

Again, gradually add the following foods one at a time in three-day increments. If you get an adverse reaction, then eliminate it for another month.

- Bread
- Corn
- Eggs
- Dairy products
- Gluten grains
- Millet
- Yeast

References

Leaky Gut Syndrome,
http://www.drkaslow.com/html/leaky_gut.ht
ml, accessed 21 Mar 11.

Adrenal Fatigue/Adrenal Exhaustion,
http://thyroid.about.com/cs/endocrinology/a
/adrenalfatigue.htm, accessed 25 Mar 11

Non-Steroidal Anti-Inflammatory Drugs,
http://en.wikipedia.org/wiki/Non-
steroidal_anti-inflammatory_drug, accessed 26
Mar 11.

The Human Digestive System,
http://www.constipationopia.com/the-human-
digestive-system.html, accessed 27 Mar 11.

Anaphylaxis,
http://www.ncbi.nlm.nih.gov/pubmedhealth/
PMH0001847/, accessed 27 Mar 11.

Cholecystokinin,
http://www.mayoclinic.com/health/drug-
information/DR600365, accessed 28 Mar 11.

Butyric Acid: an Ancient Controller of
Metabolism, Inflammation and Stress Resistance,
http://wholehealthsource.blogspot.com/2009/1
2/butyric-acid-ancient-controller-of.html,
accessed 28 Mar 11.

Parasites, http://www.cdc.gov/parasites/,
accessed 28 Mar 11.

Testing for Leaky Gut Syndrome,
http://www.leakygut.co.uk/testing.htm,
accessed 29 Mar 11.

Healing a leaky gut naturally,
http://www.stopleakygut.com/healing,
accessed 29 Mar 11.

Leaky gut syndrome treatment, http://www.ei-
resource.org/treatment-options/treatment-
information/leaky-gut-syndrome-treatment/,
accessed 29 Mar 11.

Digestion and GI Health,
http://www.womentowomen.com/digestionan
dgihealth/leakygutsyndrome-
intestinalpermeability.aspx#healingleakygut,
accessed 29 Mar 11.

Gut Dysbiosis,
http://www.regenerativenutrition.com/natural
-supplements-cure-gut-dysbiosis.asp, accessed
29 Mar 11.

Healing with probiotics,
http://www.healingdaily.com/detoxification-
diet/probiotics.htm, accessed 1 Apr 11.

How to Use a Rotation Diet, http://www.food-
allergy.org/rotation.html, accessed 2 Apr 11.

FOS -- Fructooligosaccharides,
http://www.naturaltherapypages.com.au/articl
e/FOS_Fructooligosaccharides, accessed 2 April
11.

Leaky Gut Syndrome Treatment,
http://www.ei-resource.org/treatment-
options/treatment-information/leaky-gut-
syndrome-treatment/, accessed 3 April 11.

Straight from the Leaky Gut,
http://www.hfldirect.com/index.php?main_pa
ge=index&cPath=124_188_192, accessed 3 Apr
11.

Slippery Elm to Treat Leaky Gut Syndrome,
http://mentalhealthsupportsite.com/diseases-
conditions-and-treatments/slippery-elm-to-
treat-leaky-gut-syndrome/, accessed 3 Apr 11.

Peppermint,
http://www.umm.edu/altmed/articles/pepper
mint-000269.htm, accessed 3 Apr 11.

Health Benefits of Chamomile Tea,
http://www.homeremediesweb.com/chamomil
e_health_benefits.php, accessed 3 Apr 11.

Echinacea,
http://www.umm.edu/altmed/articles/echina
cea-000239.htm, accessed 4 Apr 11.

Vitamin E,
http://www.nlm.nih.gov/medlineplus/ency/a
rticle/002406.htm, accessed 4 Apr 11.

Vitamin B-12 Shots, Injections, and Benefits,
http://www.b12shots.info/could-repairing-
your-leaky-guy-syndrome-be-the-key-to-your-
good-health/, accessed 4 Apr 11.

B12,
http://www.mayoclinic.com/health/vitamin-
B12/NS_patient-vitaminb12, accessed 4 Apr 11.

Leaky gut syndrome,
http://www.herbs2000.com/disorders/leaky_g
ut_syndrome.htm, accessed 4 Apr 11.

Managing Stress,
http://cmhc.utexas.edu/stress.html, accessed 4
Apr 11.

The Benefits of Yoga for Stress Management,
http://stress.about.com/od/tensiontamers/p/p
rofileyoga.htm, accessed 4 Apr 11.

Yoga: Tap into the many health benefits,
http://www.mayoclinic.com/health/yoga/CM
00004, accessed 4 Apr ll.

Yoga can help beat stress,
http://www.gladstoneobserver.com.au/story/2
011/04/09/yogas-happy-hormones-can-help-
beat-workplace-stres/, accessed 4 Apr ll.

Yogi, http://en.wikipedia.org/wiki/Yogi,
accessed 6 Apr 11.

Effects of stress and health on productivity,
http://www.clarityseminars.com/stress_clinical
_research.html, accessed 6 Apr 11.

What is chi gong?,
http://www.qigonghealing.com/qigong/whati
s.html, accessed 6 Apr ll.

Meditation, Take a stress-reduction break wherever you are, http://www.mayoclinic.com/health/meditatio n/HQ01070, accessed 6 Apr 11.

Basic Steps for Learning Meditation, http://www.srichinmoybio.co.uk/blog/meditat ion/basic-steps-for-learning-meditation/, accessed 7 Apr ll.

Exercise and stress: Get moving to combat stress, http://www.mayoclinic.com/health/exercise-and-stress/SR00036/NSECTIONGROUP=2, accessed 8 Apr 11.

Glutamine, http://www.whfoods.com/genpage.php?tname =nutrient&dbid=122, accessed 10 Apr 11.

Vitamin E, http://ods.od.nih.gov/factsheets/vitamine/, accessed 10 Apr 11.

Magnesium, http://ods.od.nih.gov/factsheets/magnesium/, accessed 10 Apr 11.

Zinc, http://ods.od.nih.gov/factsheets/Zinc-QuickFacts/, accessed 10 Apr 11.

Books

Lipman, Frank; Gunning, Stephanie, Total Renewal: 7 Key Steps to Resilience, Vitality, and Long-Term Health, Penguin, NYC, NY, 2004.

Lipski, Elizabeth, Leaky Gut Syndrome, Keats Publishing, Los Angeles, CA, 1998.

Rippe, M.D., James M., Your Plan for a Balanced Life, Thomas Nelson, 2008.